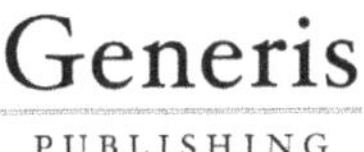

AF408120

Texts and... pretexts

Maria Dorina Pașca

Title: **Texts and... pretexts**

ISBN: 979-8-89248-986-7

Author: Maria Dorina Pașca

Cover image: www.pixabay.com

Publisher: Generis Publishing
Online orders: www.generis-publishing.com
Contact email: info@generis-publishing.com

Title: TEXTS AND. . . PRETEXTS

Author: Maria Dorina Paşca

Author: Maria Dorina Paşca

Translation: Roxana-Maria Iagăr, Mihaela- Cristina Creţu

CIP description of the National Library of Romania Maria Dorina Paşca

TEXTS AND. . . PRETEXTS / Maria Dorina Paşca.

- Târgu Mureş: Ardealul Press 2019

ISBN 978-606-8372-60-0

The translation was made with the permission of the author in the current year, 2025

(Roxana-Maria Iagăr, Mihaela-Cristina Creţu)

CONTENTS

The place and role of interactive methods in stimulating teaching activities with medical students

The teacher-student relationship may represent in certain situations the key to the realization of some didactic activities who, carried out during the appropriate pedagogical time (course and/or seminar), can determine the existence of a new psycho-pedagogical attitude and conduct, in first place, the act of teaching-learning, but also the participation and the interactive participation of the two actors directly involved in this stimulating-creative approach.

In this context, the existence of applicative exercises/play in certain disciplines of the socio sciences (in this case- medical psychology, medical sociology, physician-patient communication), determines but also values a new educational behavior, namely, communication and interrelated teacher-student vs. student-teacher.

The use of applicative exercises/play as a starting point in different knowledge dimensions can become a permanent part of university teaching activities, which appeal to the various solutions found in solving problematic situations existing in a given context. Thus, by capturing the student's attention, stimulating his thinking, imagination and volitional-emotional values, we can realize educational sequences that can and put into value, including the experiences of „freshman'' of the first year, realizing the whole in the year VI, Nelso J. R. (2014) remarks in an Indian proverb that: "Do not judge any person until you have walked for at least two months with his moccasins'', which is actually the knowledge by the teacher/magister of the student 'study and practical modality through applied educational strategies, those assimilated by the one in question.

In this context, "shoes the moccasins of student'' (metaphorically speaking) the teacher will be able to answer some questions, starting from:

- motivate or not motivate the student to attend the course and/or seminar?
- what would he want to hear from him, the student at the course and/or the seminar?
- how involved is the student in the course and/or seminar?
- how and how correctly can the student manage the knowledge assimilated to the course and/or seminars?

- is it or is it not called to the life experience of the student, in direct connection with the style and quality of his own life?

And, at the same time, the enumeration could continue important being the educational logistics applied to achieve the objectives both operational-cognitive and attitudinal-affective, so that the pedagogical time allocated, be used to the maximum by the two actors directly interested and involved: the teacher and the student vs the student and the teacher.

To make the idea outlined above plausible, we will refer directly to the disciplines to which they have applied over the years, being made today, proving their veracity in time, the applied exercises/game, being present in certain didactic sequences (of the course and/or the seminar) of the teaching-learning process, from its perspective, instructive-educational, educational highlighting your disciplines:

- Medical psychology
- Medical sociology
- doctor-patient communication

Also, both courses and the seminars have always started from their concept phase, and the interactive element/status, thus determining a new attitudinal-behavioral conduct on the part of the students, being in accordance and responding creatively to their requirements and wishes, taking into account permanently their age peculiarities, but also the sometimes pressing need to know and know themselves, overcome and surpass themselves, and performance is the certainty of complex human development.

At the same time, Berne E (2002), the first minutes were made up of those related to 'the breaking of the'' ice (accommodation, acceptance, understanding, communication, relating) so that in teaching and assimilation of new knowledge did not meet the eternal barrier from some students (this, and slides, I get bored, sleepy, it's so monotonous it does not motivate me, why I came, I do not understand, I am just a spectator, it sucks) determining and motivating him attitudinally by the appearance in the context of teaching activities, of interactive methods, they always taking into account the damage of:

- course and/or seminar topics.
- the favorable pedagogical/strategic moment in the teaching activity.
- the availability of the student to actively participate by relating to/in the teaching activity.

- the existence of feedback from the student, as a way of assessing the act of teaching-learning those taught by the teacher.
- his emotional-affective involvement during the pedagogical course and/or seminar, considering this period, in some cases. Short, the educational behavior changing both on one side and on the other.

Our educational-motivational approach considered as a tool for working in the form of interactive methods mainly - applied exercise/game, is added to it in a logical-constructive-evolutionary order and in the context of socio-human disciplines, taught, the following:

- words/words.
- proverbs and sayings.
- houghts and maxims.
- quotes.
- moral narratives.
- the therapeutic stories

Their sequence is not accidental at all, it also highlighting the element of cognition at this age (adolescence) of the student, trying to design and a future cultural approach of the medical act itself that he will carry out by not forgetting that a doctor is and always will be a fine and intellectual and cultured man of the city and not only.

Certainly, through the psycho-pedagogical exercise undertaken, it follows that its direct involvement in the academic teaching activities, transforms the act of teaching-learning into a reality of the relationship of the two actors: teacher-student vs student-teacher, learning having an interactive character and its valences determine over time, states and attitudinal-behavioral conduct, present in a certain context as a result of the ethical-moral activities and values acquired during the training in a higher education unit (medical in our case), starting from what Goethe said "If you treat an individual as he is, he will remain as he is, if it will be treated as you would like it to be or could be, it will become the desired one or the one that could be. "

So, this book is the beginning and pretext as a guide, for.

Conf. Univ. Dr Psych. Maria Dorina Pasca

Chapter 1 – WORDS

- Walk healthy!
- Go healthy!
- Be healthy!
- Stay healthy!
- To find you healthy!
- Welcome to health!
- Good I found you healthy!
- Health!
- Let's good luck and health!
- May God give you health!
- I worship with health like a green meadow!
- Go healthy!
- When I grow up, I want to be. . . a grandmother!
- Hospital food tastes like loneliness.
- I'm tired of being. sick.
- Sick of. . . unlove!

There are two kinds of pain: one that hurts you and one that changes you.

- Noise does no good, and good does not make noise.
- Not reason, but the heart knows the way.
- Sometimes you have to shut up to be heard and go to be noticed.
- The hardest disease is.
- He lost the way and the path.
- And tomorrow is another day.
- After the night, there always comes day.
- Without love and forgiveness, the patient cannot be healed.
- A full pan saturates you, and an empty pan educates you.
- Not the country needs to be changed, but our way of being.
- Heal me, O Lord, for my bones have been troubled!
- Love is friendship that caught fire!
- I've already ground a sack of speaks.
- Your name and value can never be taken away from you.

Chapter 2 – PROVERBS AND SAYINGS

- Health is a great art. (Arab proverb)
- Health is more important than religious habits. (Indian proverb)
- Health is the foundation of wealth. (Persian proverb)
- For a healthy man, every day is a holiday. (Turkish proverb)
- The doctor cures you of illness, but not of death. He is like a roof that protects you from the rain, but not from lightning. (Chinese proverb)
- Where the sun enters, the doctor does not.
- He who wakes up early reaches far.
- Mens sana in corpore sano. (A healthy mind in a healthy body.)
- Do not judge anyone until you have walked at least two months in his moccasins. (Indian proverb)
- Words are just words, without heart, they have no meaning. (Chinese proverb)
- When you have more than you need, extend the table, not the fence.
- Medicine is of two kinds: one that stimulates the strength and vitality of the healthy, and another that treats diseases. (Chinese proverb)
- A man's face is the mirror of his soul.
- A full stomach does not enjoy learning.
- You cannot straighten the world with your back.
- The eyes are the mirror of the soul.
- A known illness is half cured.
- A long illness means certain death.
- Old age does not come alone, but with many needs.
- Old age will come to ask where youth has gone.
- When you have health, guard it like something sacred.
- When you lack health, you start searching for it.
- You think he's healthy, but inside he's hollow.
- Everything hurts him, yet he considers himself healthy.
- Health gives you everything, illness takes away half.
- When the woman lies sick, the house is empty and bare.
- Illness passes from person to person, like the caterpillar from tree to tree.
- There is no illness that won't come to light.
- An inborn illness has no cure.
- Better to be healthy and poor than rich and sick.

- Everything is good and beautiful when a person is healthy.
- Anything in excess is not healthy.
- Illness enters by the cartload and leaves through the eye of a needle.
- The sick man says many things, but the doctor does what he knows.
- Health is better than all the wealth.
- In a healthy body, a healthy mind.
- Not every walnut has a good and healthy core.
- Health is better than everything.
- Health makes money, and money makes health.
- It is truly good and beautiful when a person is healthy.
- A tree with deep roots does not fear the storm.
- At a table of learning, a cartload of good behavior is required.
- Before you cut, think twice.
- Everyone should consult with themselves. (Indian proverb)
- You have won, keep going!
- You haven't won, keep going!
- Beautify the lives of others without asking for anything in return.

Chapter 3 – Reflections / Maxims:

- All bodily illnesses are caused by minds used only halfway, for it is the mind that shapes the body.
- Use your health to its limits if needed. That's why you have it. Spend it all before you die, and don't live longer than you are meant to.
- The body always ends up becoming a burden.
- Do not disdain a mild illness for which there are remedies—take the remedy.
- Do not allow the weight of your body to be great if your worth is small.
- A man's heart is his life, his prosperity, and his health.
- Even if it is little, food brings health.
- Do not build illusions for tomorrow before it comes, no one knows what troubles it may bring.
- Speak only when you are able to say something perfectly.
- The fortunate fate of a good man is given by his sharp mind.
- After sermons and defeats, people grow with more modesty and wisdom.
- There is something within each of us that is deeper than ourselves.
- We know what we are, but not what we may become.
- A great flaw: to imagine yourself as more than you are, and to value yourself less than you're worth.
- Examine yourself and you will find within a treasure which, if you know how to manage it, will produce endlessly.
- Set yourself one rule at a time, by which to guide your entire life.
- The best-conceived plans risk failing if they are not put into action immediately.
- If I don't take time to quietly reflect, I'll never hear what life is truly asking of me.
- Listen to both the youngest and the wisest, but in the end, make your own decision.
- Only those who can master themselves are truly fit to lead others.
- In the ancient temples of Greece, Aesculapius didn't speak, he listened.
- The real tragedy isn't lacking sight, but lacking vision.
- If a book sits untouched on a shelf, does it really make a difference?
- Anyone can show up, but only those who are strong enough can stay.
- Never let the chair you sit on be taller than the pile of books you've actually read.

Chapter – 4 Quotes

- No matter how you feel, get up every morning and prepare to spread your light. (Paulo Coelho – Manuscript Found in Accra)
- A woman who buries her husband is called a widow. A man left without his wife is called a widower. A child without parents is an orphan. But what do you call a father and mother whose child has died? (P. F. Thomése – Shadow Child)
- Lord, grant me the serenity to accept the things I cannot change, the courage to change the things I can, and the wisdom to know the difference. (The Serenity Prayer)

- **Three faces by Lucian Blaga:**

The child laughs:

''Wisdom and love, for me, are play!''

The young man sings:

''Play and wisdom, for me, are love!''

The old man is silent:

''Love and play are wisdom!''

- Make it mandatory that the doctor who wears a brass plate has written on it, besides the letters that show his qualification, the words:

"Remember that I too am mortal."

- Man spends ten years being a small child, unable to tell the difference between death and life. He spends another ten years learning… he spends another ten years chasing earnings and gaining wealth to live from it. He spends another ten years to reach the end of the time when his mind has reached understanding. (*Papyrus Insinger, XVII 22-23, XVIII 1-2*)

- Health is and must remain a state of psychological, physical (somatic), and social well-being of the individual, a fact which determines the existence of a balance between this and disease, the latter being seen as having the power to disrupt the harmony that makes the human being the creation of life, amplifying the desire to live, without anything that man, in his ignorance, could do to disturb it. (*Tudose Fl. - 2000*)

- We must add that what is harmful is not so much the stressful environment, but the way we approach a certain lifestyle. Stress does not come by itself, it is neither good nor bad: only its consequences on the body and psyche of an individual allow us to assess whether its overall effect is positive or negative. (Iamandescu I. B. - 1997)

- If you treat an individual as he is, he will remain as he is, but if you treat him as you would like him to be or as he could be, he will become what you desire or what he could become. (*Goethe*)

- We never understand ourselves more than when we once again have before our eyes what we did years ago, when we could look at ourselves as an object. (*Goethe*)

- No man becomes strong by reading a gymnastics manual, but by doing exercises; no man learns to judge by reading judgments written by others, but by judging himself and understanding the nature of things. (*M. Eminescu*)

- Just as the doctor does not heal the patient, but the latter heals himself under the doctor's guidance, so too the student corrects himself thanks to the teacher's guidance. (*E. Planchard*)
  God gave me a gift, and this gift is not for sale because there is no money that could pay for it. Those who take money are not doctors, and those who are doctors do not take money—everyone has a choice. (Dr. Alexandru Pesamosca - "Tata Pesi")

- Give those you love wings to fly, roots to grow, and reasons to return to where they came from. (*Dalai Lama*)

What am I / are we?

Yes, who am I / are we?

At the doorstep of an inn, a traveler addresses the woman serving customers:
- A jug of wine, beautiful lady?

- I'm not beautiful; I'm the innkeeper, she replies.

- You can be, the traveler adds. (So, you too can be anything or anyone if you truly wish for it.)

- What are you doing?

I'm waiting for myself. (*Emil Cioran*)

- The Hippocratic Oath:

"I swear! I will care for the sick for their benefit, as much as my strength and mind will help me, and I will avoid causing them any harm or injustice. "(fragment)

- Prayer of Maimonides
  "...I implore You, do not let me stray from the noble toil of aiding my fellow humans. Strengthen and fortify the powers of my body and mind so that I may always be ready to help equally the rich and the poor, the good and the bad, those who love and those who hate. Do not let me see in the most ill person anything but a fellow human being..." (fragment)

- If we consider health as a harmonious balance among various organs and functions, then illness can be seen as a disruption of this equilibrium. When we view disease as a break in the general psychophysical balance, caused by either a deficiency or an excess in the activity of a function, understanding precisely which function is altered and in what way (through excess or insufficiency) allows us to determine the most appropriate type of intervention. (P Santagostino)

- The objective of thinking is not correctness, but efficiency. To be efficient, we ultimately need to think correctly, but there's an important difference between the two. Being right means being right all the time. Being efficient means being right only at the end. (*E. de Bono*)
- There are things you know, but you don't know that you know them. When you realize what you didn't know you knew, then you'll change. *(Erickson- after Pașca M. D. -2008)*
- Remember, happiness doesn't depend on who you are or what you have; it depends solely on what you think. (*Dale Carnegie- after Pașca M. D. -2017*)
- I once asked for a bouquet of flowers and received a cactus with thorns. I was puzzled and frightened, disillusioned.

Was the world not as I believed? After a few days, unexpectedly, the cactus full of thorns… bloomed.

- - What are you?

  - How are you?

  - What are you doing?

(Questions still found today inscribed on the facade of a house in… Fălticeni, 2016)

Chapter 5 – MORAL NARRATIVES

A. From the year 1852

Health is the most precious gift on earth. As long as a person is healthy, they enjoy everything; but for the infirm, all things are bitter. Therefore, preserve your health, for if you lose it, you will not regain it. Do not strain beyond measure when lifting; do not overindulge in pleasures and frolics. If you are tired, do not drink cold water; if you are sweaty, do not go out into the cold.

Maintain cleanliness and good order in all things. Let your body be clean, your garments clean, and everything in your house clean. Where there is no cleanliness and good order, poverty and misery will soon follow.

Moderation is the best measure in eating and drinking. A moderate person lives peacefully. Therefore, do not overindulge in pleasures and comforts. Do not overdo it with food and drink. Eat as much as you like today, but you'll still be hungry tomorrow. And no matter how beautiful the clothes you wear, you will still be the same person. People judge you not by your garments, but by your good conduct.

Do what is right and fear no one.

What you learn in youth, you will find in old age.

A quiet person is pleasing to all.

Decalogue for Maintaining Health

1. Fresh and clean air
It is good to breathe.
But foul air spoils greatly
And does not bring health.
Therefore, maintain the finest
Cleanliness in the house.

2. If thirst overtakes you
Cold water is good to drink,
But even this beverage
Is good only in moderation.

3. If you're not very hungry
Do not eat just because others are eating,
And if you've had enough,
Stop eating.

4. Learn to work from a young ageAnd you will arm yourself well,
If you are diligent from youth,
You will grow up healthy.

5. Sleep
Sleep strengthens a person,
Sleep refreshes a person.
God works, He toils,
But at night, He rests.

6. Keep your body washed
And your clothing clean.
White and clean linens
Are for long-lasting health.

7. Avoid sorrow
For it shortens your life,
And also avoid sudden anger,
For it brings illness.

8. Neither too hot nor too cold
Should your dwelling be.
In winter, do not go unclothed,
And in summer, avoid overheating.

9. Protect your head from getting wet,
Your stomach from cold,
Your feet from dampness,
And your lower back from strain.

10. Refrain from all things
That are not for health;
Be moderate in all,
Fresh and in good spirits,
So you will grow healthy
And be very fortunate.

B. Present-day / In our times: Guard your heart above all else

I checked into the hospital for a routine check-up and found out I was ill.

My blood pressure was taken, and I have an extremely low level of gentleness.

My temperature was taken, and the thermometer registered 40 degrees of selfishness.

I had an electrocardiogram, and the diagnosis was that I needed several love bypasses, because my veins were blocked and not pumping blood to my empty heart.

I ended up in orthopedics; I couldn't walk alongside my brother or hug him because I had a fracture after stumbling over my vanity.

I realized I had myopia because I couldn't see beyond appearances.

They also found deafness, and the diagnosis was that I had been left alone among the empty words of each day. Pathetic, isn't it?

I also received treatment: every day, when I arrive at work, a spoonful of „Good morning!"

At each hour, a tablet of patience and a cup of tolerance.
When I get home, an injection of love,
And before bedtime, two capsules of a clear conscience. (Aurel Vâga)

Love Will Never Perish

Once upon a time, there was an island where all human feelings lived: Joy, Sadness, Wisdom, Love, and others. One day, the feelings learned that the island would soon sink, so they prepared their boats and left.

Only Love decided to ask for help.

Wealth passed by in a luxurious boat, and Love said:

-Wealth, can you take me with you?

-I can't take you; there's too much gold and silver in my boat, and there's no room for you.

Love then asked Pride, who was passing by:

-I can't help you, Love, everything here is perfect... you might ruin my boat. Love then asked Sadness, who was passing by:

-Oh, Love, I am so sad that I need to be alone.

Even Joy passed by Love, but was so content that she didn't hear Love calling.

Suddenly, a voice said:

-Come, Love, I'll take you!

It was an old man who had spoken. Love felt so grateful and full of joy that she forgot to ask the old man his name. When they arrived on shore, the old man left. Love realized how much she owed him and asked Knowledge who had helped her. When Love found out it was Time, she wondered why it was him. Knowledge, full of wisdom, replied:

-Because only Time is capable of understanding how important Love is in life. (Aurel Vâga)

Wandering Thoughts
by Octavian Paler

We've grown accustomed to living in rooms and seeing nothing but the windows
beside us.
And as we become accustomed, we forget the sun, we forget the air, we forget the
vastness... and because we lack vision, later on, we get used to not looking outside.
We get used to waking up scared because we're late.

. . . We drink our coffee in a rush because we're running behind, without looking outside;

. . . We read the newspaper on the bus because we can't afford to waste time.

We eat a sandwich because we don't have time for lunch.

We leave work in the evening.

We fall asleep on the bus because we are tired.

We have a quick dinner and then sleep without having lived the day.

We get used to thinking on behalf of those close to us:

…they'll always be there and we believe they're fine.

…We wait all day and finally hear over the phone:

-I can't come today… We'll see when we can meet… Maybe next week.

We smile at people without receiving a smile in return. We are ignored precisely when we need to be seen.

If our work is hard, we console ourselves by thinking about the weekend.

And on the weekend, we don't have much to do because we don't have money.

…We go to bed early and that's it,…because we're behind on sleep anyway.

"Death is so certain of its victory that it gives a whole life as an advantage. "

Time cannot catch us, much less stop us…

. . . Our existence passes at great speed, but as long as we are alive…

we have the opportunity to change our habits, to have a better quality of life.

…To take advantage and enjoy every breath, every heartbeat.

God provides us with all the elements to be happy, content, and grateful…

…for this gift, bestowed upon us with immense love: LIFE.

Life is not something to be saved… it must be lived TO THE FULLEST…!

The 12 Cups of Midnight

1. The first cup I raise for **health**.

…Because all the money in the world can't buy it.

2. The second cup I raise for **love**.

…Because life is given to us for love, not for hate…

3. The third cup I raise for **luck**.

…The luck of not lacking anything in life.

4. The fourth cup I raise for **dreams**.

…So that they never leave us…

5. The fifth cup I raise for **courage**.

…The courage to accept the things we cannot change…

6. The sixth cup I raise for **rediscovery**.

…Love, tenderness, and friendship help us never to be alone…
7. The seventh cup I raise for **family**.
…For the strong bonds of a united family…
8. The eighth cup I raise for **success**.
…In all our endeavors…
9. The ninth cup I raise for **peace**.
…In the world, among us, and within ourselves…
10. The tenth cup I raise for **gratitude**.
…For "BEING" every single day…
11. The eleventh cup I raise for **your imagination.**
…So I can be sure you haven't forgotten anything.
12. The twelfth cup I raise **for the most important thing…**
…The heavenly blessing of the good Lord for each day of the coming year.

Don't Ask Me to Remember
by Owen Daunell

Don't ask me to remember,
Don't try to make me understand,
Just let me rest and know you're with me,
That's enough.
Kiss my cheek and hold my hand.
If you knew how unclear everything is to me,
How sadly sick and lost I am…
All I know is that I need you,
Stay by my side no matter what,
Don't scold me, don't curse me, and don't cry.
I can't be any different, no matter how much I wish.
But you must remember that I need you.
That even the best part of me is gone…
Stay with me,
Love me.
Until the day I, too,
Will embark on the road of no return.

The Decalogue of Silence
by Rafael Noica

Be silent if you have nothing valuable to say.
Be silent when you've spoken enough.
Be silent until it's your turn to speak.
Be silent until you're prompted to speak.
Be silent when you're angry or irritated.
Be silent when entering the church so that God may speak to you.
Be silent when leaving the church so that the Holy Spirit may imprint in your mind
the things you've heard.
Be silent when you're tempted to speak.
Be silent when you're tempted to criticize.
Be silent when you have time to think before speaking.
AMEN!

The Worry Paradox

In life, there are only two things to worry about: whether you're healthy or sick.
If you're healthy, there's nothing to worry about.
If you're sick, there are only two things to worry about: whether you'll get better or
whether you'll die.
If you get better, there's nothing to worry about.
If you die, there are only two things to worry about: whether you'll go to Heaven or
to Hell.
If you go to Heaven, there's nothing to worry about.
If you go to Hell, you'll be so busy shaking hands with all your friends that you
won't have time to worry.
So why worry? (Aurel Vâga)

Learning to Be the Best
by Donna L. Clovis

Teach me to walk, and I will run.
Teach me to look, and I will see.
Teach me to hear, and I will listen.
Teach me to sing, and I will rejoice.
For what you tell me to do will be imprinted in my mind,
And the experiences you share with me, I will cherish.

What I have learned, I will value,
And by learning to fly,
I will soar!

I Can

I can overcome my fears,
I can bring food to the hungry,
I can help stop pollution,
I can give to the poor,
I can be whatever I want,
I can use my mind,
I can give advice,
I can receive,
I can behave kindly,
I can listen,
I can think,
I can teach others,
I can know,
I can give,
I can feel,
I can see,
I can.
I can.

Foundation
by Marin Sorescu

We, Ion and Ioana,
With our own strength,
Have built this sacred

CHILD

For the eternal remembrance
Of this sun
And this earth!

Chapter 6 – Therapeutic Stories

1. Lack of Communication and Connection

Give Him Your Hand!

A man had sunk into a swamp in the northern part of Persia. Only his head remained above the mire. He was shouting with all his might for help.

Soon, a crowd gathered at the scene of the accident. One person decided to try to save the poor man. "Give me your hand," he shouted. "I'll pull you out of the swamp. " But the man stuck in the mud continued only to cry out for help and did nothing to allow the other to assist him. "Give me your hand," the man pleaded several times. But the response was always just a plaintive cry for help.

Then, someone else approached and said:

"Don't you see that he will never give you his hand? You must give him your hand.

Then you will be able to save him. "

2. Personal Identity

The Teacher, a Gardener

The work of a teacher is like that of a gardener who cares for different plants. One plant loves sunlight, another prefers cool shade, one thrives in sandy soil, another in rich earth. Each requires the care that suits it best, otherwise the result will not be satisfying.

Dirty Nests

A little dove kept changing her nest. The strong smell that developed in the nests over time, was important to her. She complained bitterly about this while talking to an experienced, old, and wise dove. The latter nodded a few times and said:

"Changing your nest all the time doesn't change anything, the smell that bothers you doesn't come from the nests but from you!"

3. Inability to Set a Life Goal

The Story of Ulysses

For some time, Ulysses had been preparing to embark on a journey that would change his life. He studied several foreign languages, as well as maps that showed different parts of the world. The destination was less important; what truly interested him was to set off.

Difficulties began to arise when he went to a travel agency to book a plane ticket. The man at the counter asked him several routine questions to determine the place and time he wanted to depart.

-I don't want to go to Mexico, Greece, or Italy.

-Then where do you want to go? the clerk asked.

-I definitely don't want to go to England, Australia, or Germany.

-I'm not interested in where you don't want to go, said the increasingly impatient clerk. We're interested in where you would like to travel.

-I'm not interested in Spain or Portugal, nor India or Russia, said Ulysses.

At that moment, he realized the deadlock he was in and returned home. That night, he had a dream: he was at an airport, watching several planes take off. Suddenly, before his eyes appeared the great Lindbergh, the first pilot to cross the Atlantic in 1927, who spoke these words to him: "Planes are made to fly, it doesn't matter where.

The pilot is the one who decides where the plane will land."

Shortly after, our hero fell asleep again. In the morning, he understood the importance of knowing exactly the destination before setting out on a journey, something he still did not know.

4. Drug Addiction

The Stork's Story

A beautiful stork built her nest on the chimney of a house. From there, she could see the sky and the sun, feel the wind, and hear the sounds of the village. Unfortunately, whenever the homeowner lit the stove, all the smoke would rise directly toward our bird. At first, the stork was very bothered by the smoke, but gradually she got used to breathing the thick fumes, and her body became increasingly intoxicated. Sometimes, the homeowner would add more and more wood to the fire, making the smoke even denser.

Over time, the stork's health began to deteriorate significantly: her eyes watered more frequently, and her beautiful feathers turned darker and lost their silky texture.

The bird was losing her joy for life. Eventually, when she could no longer endure it, she decided to leave her nest. Because her wings trembled and her vision was blurred, she couldn't fly very far. She landed on a beach where some children were playing. They were surprised to see the bird and wondered what had happened to her. They decided to wash her wings and clean off the dirt. Then they fed her milk and other plants to cleanse her body of toxins.

Since their parents owned a bird cabin, they moved the stork to that place, away from smoke and sheltered from the rain. In her new home, the bird felt better with each passing day. Every morning, she thanked those who had helped her see the sun's brightness and the sky's clarity once again.

5. Quarrelsome Behavior, Irritability

The Story of Pogonici the Hedgehog

In a forest lived a hedgehog who used to pick flowers and then crush them. One day, a deer saw him picking flowers and asked why he was doing that.

Pogonici felt anger rising within him:

-Mind your own business, you're bothering me, said the hedgehog.

-But it's not right to pick flowers for no reason, they haven't done anything to you, replied the deer.

The hedgehog went on his way. At the edge of the lake, he saw a little rabbit sleeping. The hedgehog began to whistle loudly.

-Hey, can't you see I'm sleeping? shouted the rabbit, annoyed.

-I don't care, said the hedgehog, and went on his way.

The following days passed in the same manner, each day, the hedgehog felt increasingly lonely because no one wanted to play with him anymore.

One evening, while returning home, the hedgehog fell into a pit. He cried out for help in vain, for no one came.

6. The Child Who Refuses to Take Medicine

Syrupy and Little Tablet

Ionel is feeling unwell. He has a headache and a sore throat. He wishes to get better because his bicycle is waiting for him in the yard. But he can't reach it. Why? He's afraid. Of what? A dog? No! A cat? No! The hen with chicks and the rooster with spurs? No! Ionel is afraid… of medicine, and his eyes are filled with tears.

Yes, of course, he knows they are good for him, but even so, he doesn't like them, doesn't want them, and doesn't wish for them at all. And so, Ionel can't get better and, ashamed, admits that he needs help.

-Who can help me? he sighs with doubt, hoping someone will hear him.

-We can, we can, he hears a voice coming from nearby.

-Who are you? Ionel asks, looking around.

-We are Syrupy and Little Tablet, say the two from the nightstand, greeting him with a smile from cap to wrapper.

Ionel looks at them, afraid. What will they do to him? But Syrupy and Little Tablet, knowing that Ionel is scared and unwell, sit down on the little chairs next to his bed, saying:

- You know, don't be afraid of us because we will help you get better. We'll treat you with a medicinal rhyme.

Listen to us for a moment:

-I am Little Tablet,
Open your little mouth
And swallow me gently,
With a drop of Syrupy
Bravo to you, dear Ionel!

-See, it is not hard at all. We have taste, a pleasant and nice smell, we are colorful and dressed in little bottles. If you listen to us and become our friend, we will help you get back to the yard very quickly.

-And what do I have to do? asked Ionel, looking at his new friends with great trust.

-Just a little thing, just learn the poem, said Syrupy and Little Tablet cheerfully, jumping back onto the nightstand. Let's repeat it together! Shall we?

Hooray!

And the three of them began reciting the poem, so gradually, Syrupy and Little Tablet helped Ionel get better.

Where is Ionel now? Where else? In the yard, riding his bicycle. And his friends, Syrupy and Little Tablet? They sit quietly and happily in the medicine cabinet.

They are sure that Ionel has bragged about them to everyone, and that's why no handkerchief cries anymore, and no shoe sneezes. Isn't that right?

7. Stories Based on Patients' Experiences

A Glass of Milk

One day, a poor young man who sold various goods door-to-door to pay for his university studies found only a ten-cent coin in his pocket and was hungry. He decided to ask for some food at the next house. But his nerves betrayed him when a beautiful woman opened the door. Instead of asking for food, he requested a glass of water.

She thought the young man looked hungry, so she brought him a large glass of milk.

He drank it slowly and then asked:

-How much do I owe you?

-You owe me nothing, she replied. We must be kind to those in need.

-Thank you! He said.

Then, Howard Kelly left that house feeling relieved and more confident in people.

After a few years, the woman became seriously ill. The doctors in her village were worried. After a short time, they sent her to the city to Dr. Howard Kelly for a consultation.

When he heard the name of the village the patient came from, he felt a special light in his eyes and a pleasant sensation. He immediately went up from the hospital lobby to her room.

The whims of fate: it was her, he recognized her immediately. From that day on, he closely monitored the woman's case, determined to do everything possible to save her life. She had undergone open-heart surgery and was recovering very slowly.

After a long struggle, she overcame the illness. She was finally healthy. Given that the patient was out of danger, Dr. Kelly asked the administrative office to send him the bill with the total expenses for approval. He reviewed it and signed it.

Moreover, he wrote something on the edge of the bill and sent it to the patient's room.

The bill arrived in the patient's room, but she was afraid to open it because she knew she would have to work for the rest of her life to pay for such a complicated procedure.

Finally, she opened it, and something immediately caught her attention: on the edge of the bill, she read these words: "Paid in full many years ago with a glass of milk."

There is no such thing as coincidence… there is an invisible hand of destiny that gives back to each what they have given.

An Easy Recovery

The grandson of a great lawgiver, named Ghabus-Waschmgir, had fallen gravely ill. All doctors and healers had lost hope, and their remedies had been of no use. Since no one could help the sick young man, the lawgiver agreed to let Avicenna, who was only 16 years old at the time, attempt to assist him.

When Avicenna entered the palace, everyone was astonished by his courage, as he was determined to alleviate the boy's suffering, even though all the wise hakims in the country had failed.

Avicenna saw the young patient, pale and weakened, lying powerless on the bed. The man did not respond to his questions, and his relatives recounted that he hadn't spoken a word for some time.

Eventually, Avicenna raised his thoughtful brow and said, "This young man requires a different kind of treatment. To provide it, I need someone who knows the city very well, someone familiar with all the streets and alleys, all the houses, and all the people who live in them. " People were astonished: "What does curing this poor boy have to do with the alleys of our city?" they asked. But despite these doubts, they listened to Avicenna and sent him a man reputed to know the city like the back of his hand. Avicenna said to him, "Name all the neighborhoods of the city. " Meanwhile, he took the patient's pulse.

When they reached the name of a particular neighborhood, Avicenna felt the young man's pulse quicken. Then, he asked to hear the names of all the streets in that neighborhood, and upon hearing the name of a certain street, the patient's pulse quickened again. Now, Avicenna requested the names of all the alleys leading off that street. The man listed them one by one, and suddenly, upon hearing the name of one alley, the patient's pulse raced. Then, all the families living in the houses on that alley were named, and the pulse revealed which house was the one in question. When the man began to mention the names of those in the house, upon hearing the name of a young girl, the patient's pulse quickened.

Satisfied with this discovery, Avicenna commented: "Very well, everything is clear. Now I know the young man's illness and its remedy."

He stood up and said to those around:"This young man suffers from an ailment called Love. That is the root of his physical affliction. He loves the girl whose name was just mentioned. Bring her to him and betroth her to this young man!"

The patient, who had been listening to Avicenna's words with great attention and anticipation, began to blush with both embarrassment and joy. The lawgiver gave the girl in marriage to his nephew, and the young man recovered in no time.

About Me

When I was younger, I had an ear illness, mumps. No, my ears didn't grow, but I had to stay quietly at home. Where? In bed, calm and patient.

The illness passed only after two weeks, so you shouldn't be afraid.

Please don't be upset either, because I have heard it's good to have mumps when you are young. Why? Well, you are in line with all the kids, but if it comes when you are older, it is worse. I don't know why, but I will ask and tell you. (Ovidiu 10 years old)

Hope, My Story

My story isn't imaginary, it is painful. It doesn't hurt terribly, but with faith and hope, you will overcome it just like I did…

You know? Everyone around you will help you, just like they helped me. I was sick (maybe I still am a little), meaning my heart had a tiny hole. Do you think it is easy to live with something like that? But

I overcame it, and now, after the surgery, I am well, even very well. I placed my hope in the doctors, but also in the medications. And I was brave and enjoy every moment. That is how I defeated the illness.

Now, I am like all the other kids. They let me do physical education at school, I laugh a lot, and I play, play, play. How do I look? I am beautiful, strong, and... restless, but I have learned to be kind to everyone around me.

You know what I found out? They say that youth is the most beautiful memory. But is it from this story or another? I don't know, but my story is called Hope, and I wrote it for you.

Enjoy being, like me, a... fighter. (Mădălina 10 years old)

Not Hearing

One day, someone at home asked me a question, and I didn't respond. I hadn't heard it. I asked what they had asked me, but still, I couldn't hear anything.

My parents looked at me with concern, and that is when I realized something was wrong. We all decided right then that I needed a check-up. And so, I ended up at the clinic. The doctor examined my ears and asked:

-Are you scared?
-Very, I replied.
-Can you hear me?
-Yes!
-And are you less afraid now that you hear me saying there is nothing wrong?
-No, I said, and I laughed.

We all laughed because, in fact, my ears were upset with me. Why? I am a bit embarrassed to tell you, but I must.

 You see, I play music so loudly that I can't even hear the lyrics or the melody, it is just noise. And... that is how my ears punished me. Now, I know how to listen to music properly, and my family is as calm as I am.

How did I get better? With trust, courage, and by overcoming the fear of going to the doctor. (Mihaela, 10 years old)

My Flowery Scarf

I love flowers, and my scarf is adorned with them. Yes, I am 10 years old and still wear a scarf on my head. Why? Well… it takes the place of hair.

I am not joking, but you can joke about it, even though I am 10 years old, just as you will be able to. When? When you undergo radiation therapy

like I did. Don't be afraid of the treatments or the scarf! You know, boys wear caps with brims. How funny they look!

In fact, in the hospital, we recognize each other by our scarves and greet one another. We are not fearful, we are victors.

How long will I wear it? Of course, I won't wait for the flowers on the scarf to wilt and press them into a herbarium, just a few more days. Why? Well, this morning, while admiring myself in the mirror, I discovered two or three strands of hair on my head.

Hooray! Hooray! It's growing! Wonderful! That's it!

Certainly, expect me at school this fall! I will be in the fifth grade with a big surprise for you, my dear classmates.

 What is it? The flowers from my scarf, placed in… the herbarium. (Ana, 10 years old)

The Sandbox

When I was five years old, I went to the park one day with my mom. While I was playing in the sandbox, I noticed a boy about my age sitting in a wheelchair. I approached him and asked if he could play with me. Being only five, I couldn't understand why he couldn't come into the sandbox to play with me. He told me he couldn't. We talked for a while, then I took my big bucket, filled it with as much sand as it could hold, and placed it on his lap. Then, I grabbed some toys and put them there too.

My mom rushed over to me and asked:

-Lucas, why did you do that?

-I looked at her and replied:

-He couldn't come to play in the sandbox with me, so I brought the sand to him. Now we can play together in the sand. (Lucas 11 years old)

8. Offering Unconditional Help

The Man Who Had Everything

Once upon a time, there was a family that was neither rich nor poor. They lived in Ohio, in a small country house. One evening, as they sat down for dinner, there was a knock at the door. The father got up from the table and went to open it.

At the door stood an old man in tattered clothes, his pants in shreds and missing buttons. He had a basket full of vegetables. He asked if they wanted to buy some vegetables from him. They bought them immediately, wanting to see him leave as soon as possible.

Over time, they became friends with the old man. He brought them fresh vegetables weekly. They soon learned that the old man was nearly blind, suffering from cataracts in both eyes. Yet, he was so friendly that they eagerly awaited his visits and enjoyed his company.

One day, when he brought them vegetables, the old man said:

-Yesterday, I had the most blessed day! I found a basket of clothes near my house that someone had gifted me.

Knowing how much he needed clothes, the family who had made this gesture said:

-How wonderful!

But the blind old man continued:

-Yes, the most beautiful thing is that I found the family who truly needed those clothes.

Chapter 7 – Practical Exercises

1. Who Are You?

The doctor asks the child patient if they know who they are, the answer can be surprising (beetle, car, frog, Superman, princess, giant, good person, bad person). The role-playing game and the act of coming to the consultation are enlightening (the doll has a stomachache because she ate…, the bad man (drunk dad) hit me last night with the wooden spoon), allowing the child to express themselves emotionally, as they need help, understanding, and acceptance. Empathy from the doctor is very welcome.

2. Have You Spoken to What Hurts?

The child patient is asked by the doctor:

 -What hurts?
-My tummy, he replies.
-Did you talk to it?
-Uh-huh.
-And what did it say?

-That I ate too much… ice cream. (In this way, the doctor discovers the cause, already knowing the effect; this approach can be applied to any organ: hand, foot, ear, etc.).

3. The Handshake

When applied to an adolescent, a handshake from the doctor serves not only as a gesture of trust and appreciation but also allows the doctor to assess the patient's condition (dry, warm, cold, slightly sweaty, anemic, firm, limp, etc.).

4. This Is Me

The adolescent is asked to complete the following statements, focusing on elements of self-awareness:

-I like to… / I don't like to…
-I am good at… / I am not good at…
-I prefer to… / I don't prefer to…
-It is good when… / It is not good when…
-I am happy when… / I am not happy when…
 (and the statements can continue)

5. What Do I Do with My Values?

The adolescent is asked to construct a hierarchy of values or not, finding their place in:

a. **Backpack** = personal storage, the place where they keep their values and from where they take them when needed (moral values);

b. **Washing Machine** – the habit through which one "cleanses, washes" values to reuse them later;

c. **Trash Can** – the container where values that are no longer needed or are disliked are discarded;

The motivation behind these choices is already considered a step towards understanding and self-awareness.

6. Shipwreck

The adolescent finds themselves on a sea voyage and, due to a storm, must urgently abandon the ship. They are asked, as a castaway, to take with them only one object, what would it be and why? (The discussion can clarify, through the reasoning behind the choice, many of the adolescent's underlying issues)

7. How Do You Feel Today?

The doctor asks the adolescent to respond to this question through a gesture, word, facial expression, or pantomime. The initial response already reveals a certain reaction and behavior of the patient at that moment.

8. Hand Outline

The doctor may ask the child or adolescent patient to draw the outline of one of their hands on a sheet of paper. For the child, this serves as a "matching key" for the next visit to the office. For the adolescent, it's an opportunity to associate each finger with a joy and/or a sorrow. The directions stemming from this exercise can be very insightful. (Pay attention to nonverbal communication)

9. The Storyteller's Chair

In front of the participants (students), there is a chair called the storyteller's chair. The person invited, willing, or chosen to sit on this chair will share something special that happened on that particular day. The audience is allowed to ask the storyteller three questions, which may or may not be related to the story told. The storyteller is obliged to answer them. This exercise helps in working on the "fear of public speaking"

10. Strengths and Weaknesses

The subject is asked to identify their strengths and weaknesses in relation to:

- a given problem situation;
- their own person;
- a clinical case under discussion;

with the aim of assessing the ability to have an opinion and to argue the points presented.

Additionally, elements of self-awareness come into play, their impact being significant when making decisions.

(example:)

- problem/situation: _____________________

- strong points: _______________________

- weak points: _______________________

11. Hug Me

The doctor may, at a certain moment, hug the patient, and vice versa, thus conveying a positive, friendly, and encouraging message, serving as both a verbal and nonverbal communication element.

12. Unlimited Possibilities

Participants are asked to express themselves as thoroughly as possible regarding one of the following questions:

- What is the most surprising thing you did this week or today?
- If you could do only one thing today, what would it be and why?
- What would you do if you could do anything?
- What did you enjoy most out of everything you did today or this week? Tell us about it and explain why.
- If you were to live on a deserted island for an entire year, what would you take with you to avoid boredom, and why?
- What do you think is the greatest job in the world, and why?
- What are you best at, and how do you feel when you are engaged in that activity?

The exercise can be continued with other prompts from the participants, including the use of negation (e. g., "What wouldn't you do...").

13. Complete the Verse

Participants are asked to complete the verse with one or two words:

a. I am...
I wonder...
I hear...
I want...
b. I understand...
I say...
I hope...
I am...

c. I pretend…
I feel…
I touch…
d. I am worried…
I cry…
I am…

14. The Decalogue of Communication

1. You cannot not communicate.
2. To communicate requires self-awareness and self-esteem.
3. To communicate requires understanding the needs of the other person.
4. To communicate requires knowing how to listen.
5. To communicate requires understanding messages.
6. To communicate requires providing feedback.
7. To communicate requires understanding the processual nature of a relationship.
8. To communicate requires knowing how to express your feelings.
9. To communicate requires accepting conflicts.
10. To communicate requires taking responsibility for resolving conflicts.

15. Rules of Communication

- Every opinion must be listened to;
- No one is interrupted;
- All questions have their purpose;
- No one is ridiculed;
- Everyone has the right not to participate actively;
- No one is criticized or moralized;
- Everyone has the right to be heard;
- No one is blamed;
- No one is judged or labeled;
- No one monopolizes the discussion;
- No one is obliged to express their point of view.

16. The Cutlery

Participants are asked to figuratively choose one of the five pieces of cutlery: spoon, fork, knife, teaspoon, and ladle, and to explain why they chose that particular one over the others. Discussions may reveal that certain traits are reflected in the personality of the chooser.

(Example: knife—sharp, direct; ladle—generous, extroverted, etc.)

17. Do You Like Your Name?

Conducted both in groups and individually, participants (students) are asked to refer to their given name, reminding them that they were not asked for their preference, but their parents chose it, based on certain criteria or not. Each person will express their opinion and make comments about their first name whether they accept it or not, whether they identify with the person whose name they happen to bear, justifying the position they adopt.

The subject is then asked to choose a desired name themselves, to mention the choice made and whether they identify with it or not, now expressing the desire to change it or not.

18. Dialogues

Compose a dialogue between a:

- doctor and patient vs. patient and doctor;
- hospital porter and relative/visitor;
- bandage and wound;
- medical instruments and nurse;
- hospital room and hospital bed;
- elevator and elevator operator;
- stretcher and patient;
- health and illness;
- life and death;

(Example: Life and Death:

Death:

- I have come!

Life replies:

- Too soon!)

19. The Waiting Game

This can be played individually or in groups, asking participants/students to mimic the state of stress or waiting, using facial expressions and gestures, in settings such as:

- doctor (hospital, medical office);
- pharmacy;
- dentist (office, waiting room);
- reception (taking a number).

Each behavior is then discussed, explaining the attitude and/or conduct exhibited at that moment.

20. The Walk

Subjects walk in an allocated space (classroom, auditorium, etc.) without knowing or communicating with each other. At a certain point (a clap from the game leader), they will stop, shake hands, greet each other, say their first names, and exchange a few words with those in front of them at that moment. At another clap from the game leader, they will resume walking, then socialize with others at the next signal. It is important not to stop at the same people but to communicate with as many as possible.

21. The Blank Sheet

A large sheet of paper is presented to the participants, and each subject is asked to describe "what they see" at that moment on the blank sheet in front of them. The reasoning behind their observations can serve as a starting point for understanding and engaging with the respective subject.

22. The Word Game

In front of the audience, a word is presented, and each participant is asked in turn to make an association with the given word. This can lead to a discussion about the choices made (e. g., white = snow, hospital, bedsheet, saint, wall, immaculate, winter, diabetes, sugar, bride, etc.).

23. Who am I?

Each participant will need to identify as many terms as possible that characterize themselves. This will help them understand how they form and develop their own identity.

I am: -

24. If-then, but…

This game discusses how a person gets involved when they have to make a major decision, how they support it, and how doubt and suspicion arise.

The pro and con arguments will be enlightening, and their reasoning leads over time to arguments and opinions that have the certainty of value:

-If:
-Then:
-But:
(Example: medical diagnosis)

25. The Cluster

On the board, the game leader writes a word, asking participants to find synonyms, and then for each found synonym, to find others, so that the resulting configuration resembles a cluster of grapes.

(Example: health)

Health – well-being – abundance:
- job
- home
- car
- children
- luck
- happiness
-Calm
-Love

Student:
- Young
- Teenager
- Away from home
- Fun
- Money
- Free
- Without control
- Tuition
- Budget
- No money

Exams:
- Failed
- Passed
- Retakes

26. Choose

Students participating in the game are asked to choose between two piles located on either side of the road (the road is drawn on the board): one marked with a plus sign (+) and the other with a minus sign (−).

They will justify:

- which one they chose and why?
- the similarities between them
- the differences between them.

27. Correlate

Draw the words that express for you: loneliness, wisdom, happiness, old age, youth, fear, love, life, death, home, hospital.

28. The Cycle of Life

Participants (students) are asked to imagine their future at the ages of: 18, 30, 40, 50, 60, 75, and beyond. The explanations of their aspirations and motivations, supported by arguments, are interesting and will be discussed.

29. Turning Negation into Affirmation

For those who are shy, introverted, have complexes, or are pessimistic, this exercise teaches something else: confidence, self-image, and self-esteem, which are at the forefront of interventions concerning self-awareness. That is: I am not / I don't know / I don't understand, but… (example: I am not bold, although I would like / wish to have the courage to speak with my colleagues / in public.)

30. Together

The group (students) is in motion (walking), and at the suggestion of the game leader, they will form groups based on:

- happy/sad
- good/bad
- rich/poor
- budget/tuition
- girls/boys

31. In Your Shoes

Played in pairs, participants are asked to exchange accessories, gloves, vests, caps, etc, and then are questioned about whether they feel comfortable in/with the borrowed items and why or why not, and how it feels to be "in someone else's shoes."

32. The Cube

Students are asked to devise a cube-type algorithm-six sides- to describe an action, a term, a state, an emotion, or a phenomenon. Given that the cube has six sides, each will focus on:

- description
- comparison
- association
- analysis
- application
- argumentation
The cube can be "played" either by:

- a group of six students, each representing a "side
- six distinct groups, each group representing a "side"

If played by forming "six faces," each group will designate a leader to support/present and justify the points made in their speech.

33. The Thinking Hats

Students are grouped into six working sequences, each being called a "hat" and having a specific color. Based on the color of the hat, the group will intervene, targeting the problem situation under discussion or argue a cognitive sequence, a quote, a reflection, a proverb, etc. The important aspect is the student's involvement and argumentation at that moment. The thinking hats are identified as follows:

1. **Blue Hat** = is the leader and conducts the activity, being responsible for controlling the discussions, drawing conclusions - **clarifies and chooses the correct solution**
2. **White Hat** – Possesses information regarding the topic under discussion, makes connections, provides raw information as received – **informs**.
3. **Red Hat** – Expresses emotions, feelings, upset towards encountered individuals, does not justify – **says what they feel**.
4. **Black Hat** – Is the critic, presents possible risks, dangers, mistakes in proposed solutions, expresses only negative judgments – **identifies errors**.
5. **Green Hat** – Offers alternative solutions, new, innovative ideas, seeks alternatives (what needs to be done?) – **generates new ideas**.
6. **Yellow Hat** – Is the creator, symbol of positive and constructive thinking, optimistically explores possibilities, creates the ending – **effort brings benefits.**

34. The Frisco Method

It is a problem-solving technique that involves participants (students) interpreting specific roles.

 The process includes:

- Identifying the problem.
- Assigning roles and forming groups:
  • C = Conservative; • E = Exuberant; • P = Pessimist; • O = Optimist;
- Debating the problem through the perspectives of C, E, P, and O.
- Systematizing ideas.
- Drawing conclusions about the proposed solution.

(Example: students and exams)

- Hospital-acquired infections.
- Doctor-patient communication.
- Communicating a diagnosis.

35. The Mosaic Method

This method is based on cooperative learning through group interdependence and the exercise of expertise in completing a learning task. The objective is to document and present the results of independent study to others, becoming an expert on the studied topic.

The steps include:

- Establishing the main topic and dividing it into four or five subtopics,
- Organizing learning groups,
- Forming expert groups,
- Initial team learning activities,
- Evaluation

36. Synthesizing

Is a method of reflection on a subject that involves a procedural approach, aiming to develop thinking processes by deepening the proposed topic through group or pair work. The steps begin with:

- Organizing into pairs/groups;
- Communicating the learning task;
- Working independently;
- Working in pairs/groups;
- Whole-class activity;

37. Knowledge and Involvement

Students are given a worksheet containing three sections, labeled:

- I know;
- I want to know;
- I have learned;

They are asked to complete the first two sections with the idea that:

-I know (they have knowledge about the subject)
-I want to know (they wish to acquire knowledge)

At the end of the learning activity, they will complete the third section based on the new knowledge acquired: I have learned.

(Example: communication, patients, diagnosis, illness, health, treatment, etc.)

38. What Color Are Your Emotions?

In a group or individually, students are asked to associate the emotions they experience or express with a color, so they can answer the question: What color are your emotions? They are then asked to justify their choice, leading to a new decoding of certain personality traits.

39. Your Business Card

Students are asked to design their own business card, starting from the perspective of their. . . future, explaining:

- the choice they made / their specialization;
- personalization;
- graphics;

40. The Statues

This game can be played in pairs and/or groups, where participants/students are asked to create a statue or a group of statues based on a given theme (for example: stress, depression, emotion, joy, etc.). Once the work is completed, it will be analyzed by the others, who will justify the choice of title.

The roles can then be switched (the sculptor becomes the "material" and vice versa).

41. You Are a Geometric Shape

Participants (students) are asked to group themselves, on command, into a specific geometric shape (for example: circle, square, rhombus), ensuring the accuracy of the shape (sides, angles). This activity can be done with the whole group (more than 20 people) or in smaller groups.

42. Butterfly or Beetle?

Participants (students) are asked to choose, for a moment, what they would like to be. After making their choice, they are asked whether they could kill a butterfly or a beetle.

This is followed by discussions about good and evil, life and death, as well as the responsibility one assumes when deciding to let someone live or die. If participants refuse, in the second round, to reverse their roles (butterfly-beetle, beetle-butterfly), the game can still continue without the participants' identities, acknowledging their refusal to accept a certain role.

43. Seven from One... Knowledge

The group of students is asked to find answers to the following questions, such as:

- **Who?** (the person);
- **What?** (the subject);
- **Where?** (the place);
- **When?** (the time);
- **How?** (the manner);
- **How much?** (the quantity);
- **Why?** (the motivation);

The topics can vary, for example: communication, medication, medical consultation, etc. Through such an analysis process, the goal is

To observe how the topic or subject in question is percieved and understood, managing to comprehend and/or resolve the problem-situation at hand.

44. Observation Sheet

Students are asked to individually observe the activity, environment, and atmosphere in a medical office, clinic, and/or hospital (public or private), without revealing that they are medical students (evaluation under. . . cover).

They will then be asked to describe everything they observed, noting details based on the following questions:

1. What did you like?
2. What didn't you like?
3. What would you change?
4. How did you feel as a patient? Why?

This minimal guided observation will help the student become aware of, and take responsibility in certain situations, regarding the role of the doctor, as well as the importance of the place where the doctor carries out their activity.

45. The 3-2-1 Technique

After completing the activity, students must specify:

- **Three new terms** they acquired during that activity;
- **Two ideas** they would like to learn more about or continue studying;
- **One skill** they believe they have acquired or improved during that activity.

46. The R. A. I. Method (Respond, Choose, Ask)

After the teaching activity is completed, students are asked to use some of the following questions:
- What do you know about…?
- What is the importance of the fact that…?
- What questions do you have regarding…?
- What did you find most difficult about…?
- What are the requirements of the fact that…?
- What other knowledge can you connect this information to…?
- How do you justify the fact that…?

47. Role-Playing Game "At the Doctor's"

Students are asked to choose characters from among themselves, such as: the doctor, the patient (considering age characteristics), the nurse, and the parents/relatives where applicable.

Practically, a part of the classroom becomes a medical office, and the characters take on their roles.

It is interesting to observe how closely our role-play resembles reality. At the end of the game, discussions take place regarding communication and the relationships between the characters.

The game is engaging and enjoyable, often including comedic moments, but also revealing certain communication gaps that need to be addressed.

48. Gathering Troubles

The game leader asks the participants/students to place everything negative for them (thoughts, emotions, worries, troubles, etc.), metaphorically speaking, into the palms of his hands. After collecting everything from everyone, the leader walks to the window, opens it... and "releases everyone from their troubles."

The game is effective and welcome, as it creates a sense of removing obstacles that stand in the way of success.

49. His Fingers

By looking at the fingers of one hand (either right or left), we should give them proper significance in our communication with an autistic patient, knowing that for them:

• **Thumb** = What do I do? (Where do I start?)
• **Index finger** = How do I do it? (The strategies used)
• **Middle finger** = Where do I do it? (The place of action)
• **Ring finger** = When do I do it? (The timing of the activity)
• **Little finger** = Who, with whom do I do it? (What resources I use)

50. Role-Playing Game – "The Tree"

Individually or in a group, this game aims to externalize emotional experiences as well as feelings of frustration.

The subject (or subjects) is asked to be a ''tree'', to behave accordingly, to live its complicated life, to move, to wither, to rejoice, to cry with it.

They must talk to: the leaves, branches, trunk, roots, and birds, all of which will question and help them. How do you feel as a tree? What is it like to be a tree?

51. Yes-No

This game is played in pairs. The rule is that while they can move freely, argue, speak loudly or softly, they are only allowed to use two words in their communication: "yes" and "no", expressing themselves with as much personality and expressiveness as possible.

The game ends when... the partners decide.

BIBLIOGRAPHY:

1. Berne, E. (2002) – *The Psychology of Human Relationships*, Amaltea Publishing House, Bucharest
2. Blaga, L. (1982) – *Poems*, Cartea Românească Publishing House, Bucharest
3. Coelho, P. (2012) – *Manuscript Found in Accra*, Humanitas Publishing House, Bucharest
4. Iamandescu, I. B. (1997) – *Medical Psychology*, Infomedica Publishing House, Bucharest
5. Manes, S. (2008) – *83 Psychological Games for Group Facilitation*, Polirom Publishing House, Iaşi
6. Nelson, J. R. (2014) – *Counseling Manual*, Trei Publishing House, Bucharest
7. Paşca, M. D. (2017) – *Identities of Psychonutritional Counseling*, University Press, Târgu Mureş
8. Paşca, M. D. (2019) – *The Story in the Doctor-Patient Relationship*, Ardealul Publishing House, Târgu Mureş
9. Paşca, M. D. (2012) – *Communication in the Doctor-Patient Relationship*, University Press, Târgu Mureş
10. Paşca, M. D. (2008) – *The Therapeutic Story*, V & Integral Publishing House, Bucharest
11. Paşca, M. D. (2007) – *New Perspectives in Medical Psychology*, University Press, Târgu Mureş
12. Paşca, M. D. (2007) – *Psychological Counseling in the University Environment*, Ardealul Publishing House, Târgu Mureş
13. Paşca, M. D., Benga, E. (2016) – *Occupational Therapies and Combined Arts – Creative Landmarks*, University Press, Târgu Mureş
14. Paşca, M. D. (2018) – *Therapy Through Theatre*, Ardealul Publishing House, Târgu Mureş
15. Peseschkian, N. (2005) – *Oriental Stories as Tools in Psychotherapy*, Trei Publishing House, Bucharest
16. Peseschkian, N. (2009) – *Psychotherapy of Everyday Life*, Trei Publishing House, Bucharest
17. Râzuş, P. (1974) – If You Can Laugh, Then Laugh (Proverbs and Sayings from Banat), Facla Publishing House, Timişoara
18. Shaw, G. B. (1989) – Aphorisms, Paradoxes, Reflections, Albatros Publishing House, Bucharest

19. Tudose, Fl. (2000) – A Modern Approach to Medical Psychology, Infomedica Publishing House, Bucharest
20. The Book of Popular Wisdom (1974) – Minerva Publishing House
21. The Free Word (2018, 2019) – Collection, Târgu Mureş
22. Proverbs (1999), Emia Publishing House, Deva
23. Dictionary of Romanian Proverbs (2003), All Publishing House, Bucharest
24. Romanian Legends for the First Grade of Elementary Schools (1852 – Samuil Andrievici) – Transcription by Maria-Dorina Paşca (2017), Renaşterea Publishing House, Cluj-Napoca

www.ingramcontent.com/pod-product-compliance
Lightning Source LLC
Chambersburg PA
CBHW061640130726
47996CB00003B/1381